7 DAYS OF MEDITATION

TO BALANCE YOUR CHAKRAS

Written by
Celestine Moore

Copyright © 2023 all rights reserved.

Written by Celestine Moore

7 Days of Meditation To Balance Your Chakras - First Edition 2023.

All rights reserved. No part of this publication may be reproduced, distributed, or transmitted in any form or by any means, including photocopying, recording, or other electronic or mechanical methods, without the prior written permission of the publisher, except in the case of brief quotations embodied in critical reviews and certain other noncommercial uses permitted by copyright law.

For permission requests, write to the publisher, addressed "Attention: Permissions Coordinator," at the address below:

Permissions@sycwp.com

Published by So You Can Write Publications.

ISBN-13: 978-1-7376084-3-1

www.sycwp.com

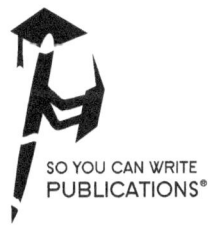

CONTENTS

Introduction	7
Sunday – Root Chakra	21
Monday – Sacral Chakra	29
Tuesday – Solar Plexus Chakra	39
Wednesday – Heart Chakra	47
Thursday – Throat Chakra	57
Friday – Third eye chakra	65
Saturday – Crown Chakra	73
Conclusion	81
Acknowledgments	86
Dedication	87

INTRODUCTION

Peace and blessings. I hope this book reaches you in great spirits and with an open mind. My intention is for this book to guide and inspire you on your meditation journey by explaining simple analogies, thoughts, and ideas that can help you understand the simplicity of meditation, regardless of how experienced you are. I want this small book to be used as one of many tools to help focus yourself mentally, physically, and spiritually while meditating.

Throughout each chapter I will explain the purpose of each of the 7 main chakras within us and how each chakra can correlate to a specific day of the week. In a nutshell, our 7 chakras are the main energetic focal points that help us to become a balanced, well-rounded human being. Each chakra is in a specific spot along our core and each one holds specific characteristics that are different but necessary. Understanding the meaning of each chakra can help us navigate in life more effectively. Below is an image breakdown for each Chakra and it's corresponding color:

THE SEVEN CHAKRAS

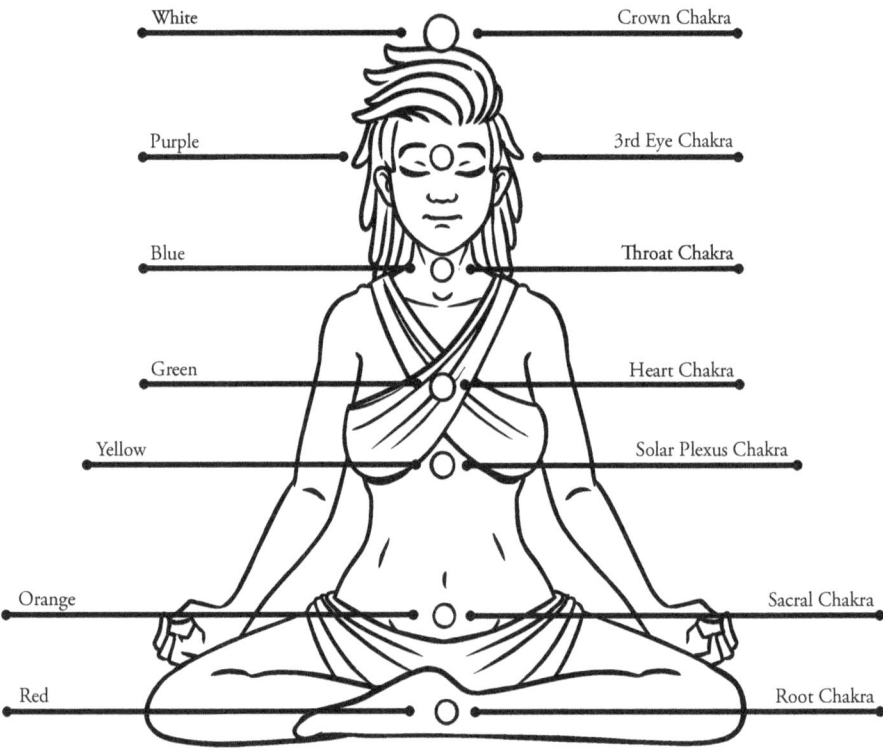

In the following chapters, I will explain more in depth the characteristics of each chakra and offer a meditation analogy, thought, or idea that can be used to help you balance that specific chakra.

A little disclaimer and background about myself: I meditate about 3-5 days a week at 20 minutes per "session" to balance my emotions and prepare for the day ahead. By staying consistent with practicing meditation for over 10 years, I've learned some things and decided to share those things to whoever wants to read about them. I feel that my perspective on meditation and my way of explaining it is unique and can help others understand meditation better. Overall, I want this book to be practical and easy to understand for regular people. I'm not emphasizing a one-size-fits-all perfect way to meditate, but I want everyday people to realize the importance of meditating however they choose to – as long as it's beneficial for you.

My meditation journey started in 2012, at a time when life was starting to get real for me. I was in my last semesters of college, pregnant, working 2 jobs, and still trying to understand how life works. This "perfect" world that I thought existed for whoever puts work in was becoming a façade and I realized that life was a bit more challenging than what I expected. Over time, I started hearing about the benefits of meditation for our health, happiness, efficiency, and overall well-being, but never took it seriously – I never needed to, I remember my first experience meditating at my elementary school (Lloyd Street, Milwaukee WI) in 1st and 2nd grade with the assistance of my amazing Art teacher Ms. Gaborsky (RIP). I stopped after that, when I felt life was positioning me between a rock and a hard place emotionally and mentally, I made the conscious decision to start practicing meditation again to see what changes can possibly happen in my life, or to myself – if any, so it wouldn't hurt to try. I felt that I had nothing to lose by meditating and there's even a chance that meditation might change my life and I might enjoy it and teach others ☺.

Through self-teaching, studying, and constant practice, I've learned different ways to relax my body and control my mind to keep myself calm and collected during most stressful situations. I started to understand the power of the imagination and visualization and knew that whatever our mind thinks about for a long enough period of time, will attached the correct emotions to our thought(s), then our body will subconsciously do the work to manifest it, which helps to shape our lifestyle. Imagining and becoming our better selves for the future, the person who we aspire to be is imperative for our well-being and evolution both individually and collectively. When we focus on our higher self, we can operate at a higher frequency and not live buried under the lower levels or the details of life which can be a distraction most times.

If we can be honest, I'm sure we would agree that this world has been changing quickly within a short time. Whether that's a good or bad thing is a personal choice, I'm sure everyone can agree that this world is not the same as it once was just a few years ago. We can also agree that there may be a lot of people who could have developed some form of undiagnosed culture shock or post-traumatic stress disorder (PTSD) from these drastic changes in their lives. Even before major events started to shift, a lot of our everyday lives have already been filled with different challenges that we've had to take care of and maintain. Challenges with our family, friends, neighborhood, school, work, and even ourselves have already been constant, so any added challenges to our lives can be overwhelming at times. Because of that, it's important (and perfect timing) to find ways to cope with these new changes and emotions within us now.

Although meditation is a great way to decompress yourself and that's what I'm advocating in this book, it's not the only way. Other practices such as sound therapy, exercising, journaling and gardening are other great examples of activities to help you understand and appreciate yourself and life better - find out which one or combination works best for you.

No two days are the same; tasks accumulate, plans are made, people are met, and life changes by the second. Every day is a challenge, so you deserve at least a few minutes to relax your heart, mind, and body periodically so that you can handle those challenges. We all need time to disconnect from the busyness of life to be with ourselves and feel our feelings naturally as they flow to understand them better. Life will still happen afterwards, so it's best for you to handle yourself and your well-being first. I recommend spending 10-20 minutes every few days a week, but it's all dependent on your time commitment and what's comfortable for you.

Time and practice are the only things that will strengthen any skill, and meditation is no different. Just like riding a bike or cooking, once you learn the basics, it will become easier each time. Understand that nothing and no one is perfect, and there will be days where your mind can't focus or your body won't cooperate, similar to riding a bike on a rocky trail or cooking with very few ingredients, you won't have it together every time, but still practicing under those stressful conditions will strengthen your ability.

It'll be a good idea to document (journal) the shift in your feelings and emotions during this time if you're beginning your meditation journey – I provided space at the end of each chapter to jot down any thoughts or feelings you may experience (preferably with a pencil). After meditating regularly, you may notice that the people or things that usually upset you may not be a big deal anymore and you may be more understanding of others.

You may become more conscious of the thoughts and actions you do and choose the ones that will be best for you and others. Everyone feel things differently, and although you cannot control the outside world, you can control your inner self and how you respond to those situations; that's one of our many superpowers that we've been equipped with.

Going within yourself to find calmness, understanding, and truth helps a lot with personal healing and growth in this new world that we're entering. Finding time daily to silence your mind and listen to your higher self is a lifelong benefit to you and others around.

Our higher selves automatically know what we need in life so when we take time to hear that voice, we can save ourselves a lot of time by avoiding potential mistakes in the future. Listening to our inner voice allows our "gut" feeling, or our intuition to become clear.

It's exciting to know that we can continuously grow to understand ourselves on a deeper level – there's no limit to how deep we can go within ourselves. We must understand that our actions are based on our emotions, and emotions fluctuate, it's always in motion, so there may be emotions we don't understand yet. Depending on the circumstances, your health, the environment, recent conversations, etc. Will determine your current emotional state so don't expect yourself to stay steady all the time.

When you choose to meditate, you are indirectly giving yourself permission to take a step back from the busyness of life to nurture yourself – to fill your cup. You can't pour into anyone else's cup if yours is empty – you can't even use your own water if there's none in the cup. It's important that you are intentional about giving yourself permission and acceptance to care for yourself for a few minutes a day without feeling guilty or that you're missing out on things by doing so. Verbally saying to yourself affirmations that nurture your body, mind, and soul is a great way to program your mind before, during, or after your meditation. As you continue meditating, you'll experience the results of taking care of your inner self first, then you'll realize that the same energy of taking care of your inner self will radiate in areas outside of yourself.

With this fast-paced, internet driven world that we've been accustomed to living in, there are a lot of distractions being pushed on us, so being alone with our thoughts can be uncomfortable at times – we're used to being entertained all the time. There also may be past trauma that was never addressed, so being alone with your own thoughts may bring up uncomfortable thoughts and emotions that were never resolved. Those emotions can be scary so it's important to give yourself permission to tap into your thoughts if your mind takes you there…through the good, the bad, and the ugly.

Understand that no one has control over what you say, how you feel, and how you respond to things. That's another superpower that we are equipped with; we make the final call in our lives. The same way we allow great things to happen (like reading this book… appreciate it!). That is the exact same way we allow bad things to happen or continue to happen in our lives…by our choices.

Our responsibility is to ourselves first, so we must make sure that we are only allowing what's best for us by any means necessary. Also, we must hold ourselves accountable for treating each other right as well as hold others accountable for treating us right.

As humans living on earth, I don't think we will ever fully understand how life works no matter how old we get. There's always something new to learn. Life has a sly way of throwing curve balls to interrupt the normal process of living. Those curve balls should be a reminder for us to step back and reassess what we've been doing and what needs to change – in other words, these curve balls or "suffering" can sharpen our sword.

Over time, we've become obsessed over the idea that we should always be "on" nonstop. Always going, working, doing. A lot of us take pride in working 60, 70, 80 hour weeks with little time to sleep, eat properly, or think clearly. Although it's good to be active and productive, over-exerting ourselves can wear our bodies down prematurely. If we slow down DOING too much and focus more on BEING, like the human BEINGS we are…I feel that our lives will start aligning in the direction they need to go.

I believe we have everything our bodies need within to heal from anything, we just haven't been taught how to use it. This powerhouse of a human body we live in is a magnificent, thinking, moving, self-healing, sun soaking machine that can do whatever our minds decide. We can control the thoughts in our mind, and we have what it takes within us to feel every emotion that passes through us, whether it's being extremely happy, excited, joyous, sad, angry, regret or many more. Our feelings are a reaction to what's happening around us, so every feeling in our body is meant to be felt – whether it be good or bad. If a feeling wasn't supposed to be felt, then it wouldn't exist, and you wouldn't feel it. So, as you read through the chapters ahead, try to embrace all the feelings and emotions that pass through.

THE HOW TO'S

Learning how to meditate seems like it should come naturally, but for most people it doesn't. It takes consistency and actual concentration from you. You can't fake the level of awareness you put into your inner self and thoughts. Meditation requires you to be real with yourself and hold yourself accountable to how serious you want to take it. Your mind will challenge you with thoughts from all over the place but concentrating on one thing can eliminate those distractions. Here are some quick tips to help you along your meditation journey:

- Eat healthy, exercise regularly, and spend time in nature.

- Make sure you are sitting or lying comfortably, with a straight back.

- Take slow deep breaths throughout the meditation, taking in as much oxygen as a good yawn. This helps your body relax and find its natural rhythm.

Concentrate heavily on things such as your heartbeat, breathing, or sounds around you while meditating. These tips may sound simple, but when it's applied, your body will become primed to practice meditation easily. Just remember - it's all up to your willingness and the effort you put in. Follow this simple ritual to help you meditate each day:

Choose a comfortable space in your house. Make sure that it is clean and uncluttered, and that you will not be disturbed. Sit comfortably, in a relaxed position. Either close your eyes or choose an object to focus on. If you're choosing an object, gaze at that object, at the same time allowing yourself to become aware of your breathing. Don't change the breathing, just watch it as it comes and goes. You may feel like taking a deep breath – and if you do, you may notice that the whole body relaxes a little as you exhale.

If you feel like closing your eyes at any point, that is fine.

Now feel the contact of your body with the floor, the cushion or the chair where you are sitting. Check out your shoulders – are they tense? Let them relax. Make whatever adjustments you need to make so that your body is comfortable, and then go back to being aware of your breathing.

SUNDAY – ROOT CHAKRA

SERVANT AND ROYALTY IN ONE

"Oh lord, I'm the rookie and the vet" – Drake

OVERVIEW

Sundays are a great day to start meditating because it's the beginning of the week and it can be the start to new goals. Sundays usually correlates to a day of relaxing and preparing for the week ahead so meditating today will clear your mind to do those things. Using this day to become aware of both the bigger picture of your life as well as the details can help you set the tone for the rest of the days, weeks, months, and even years ahead.

Ground and center your energy by focusing on your first chakra today. This helps you prepare for the coming week. Release anything from the past week and start fresh. This is also a great day to relax and spend time with your loved ones.

This first day of the week - Sunday is correlated to our first chakra - the root chakra. The root chakra is located at the base of our spine and has connections with the Earth, physical survival, feelings of safety, and security vs. fear. When our root chakra is balanced, we feel like our lives are on track and everything will be okay – even if it doesn't physically look so at the moment. Our basic needs are met when our root chakra is balanced. There's a certain calmness in our heart that's priceless when our root chakra is balanced.

We begin our lives developing the root chakra's energy for the first 7 years. Our root chakra is the energy that grounds us and "bring us down to Earth" whenever our head is up in the clouds from our ego. The energy from our root chakra is also what keeps us alive and instinctively knowing how to protect ourselves in times of fear or life-or-death (fight/flight).

The purpose of this meditation below is to help picture yourself as both the Rookie and the Vet, or Royalty and Servant at the same time. As royalty (Vet), you have complete control over your kingdom (life) and as the servant, you make sure the people, places, and things in between are loved and being maintained and taken care of.

MEDITATION

I understand and sympathize with all humans because I know that every race has went through struggles and setbacks throughout history. However, for African Americans (because that's the only race I'm experiencing and living through), let's start by understanding that throughout generations of slavery, torture, abortions, genocides, and other destructive things that have traumatized many humans and could've ended our existence; we've been fortunate to make it this far. There's no doubt that every one of our lineages has stood the test of time.

You are royalty in the presence of other royalty on this Earth – no matter what level in life you're on. You and the gifts you possess have a purpose and designated spot on this earth which means there's work to do to manifest and experience those gifts. We've already earned our crowns and titles as royalty by overcoming the odds to be on this earth right now. Now we need to cultivate the seeds that's been planted within us so that we can share them with the rest of the world.

When you meditate today, imagine yourself as royalty, and picture yourself sitting on your personal throne. The throne is your essence. The throne is your truth…it holds the reason behind what you're here for, it knows the reason why you're taking up space. Your essence is who you really are – your truth – and it's equipped with everything you need within to grow into the person you're meant to be. Your essence holds peace, and it gravitates towards people or situations that makes you and others better.

After a few deep breaths to relax your body, also imagine mini versions of yourself taking care of every function in your life such as money, family, health, etc. GRACEFULLY – your personal servants. In your vision, you see each version of yourself working diligently to keep your temple running smoothly. Similar to a car and all its parts - each piece has a place in the car; if one part is off, it makes the "whole" car less efficient, therefore, the car won't be able to move the way it should.

Your servant self, the physical lower self is meant to serve – whether it's serving yourself or others to be better. Your servant self doesn't worry whether people appreciate or reciprocate the good deeds you put out there, the people are going to receive it from you whether they like it or not. That doesn't mean you need to be a doormat, so it's good to understand where to continue serving and where to stop. Although our royal self is a visionary and is focused on the bigger picture, he/she still finds joy in the small acts of kindness and understand that our good works are always being brought back to us and being accounted for.

When you meditate today, feel the inside and outside of your body confidently sitting on your gold plated, high-energy throne. You feel calm and comfortable yet alert and present. You are naturally able to ease every part of your muscles and release the weight of your body onto your throne. You feel confidence radiating out of your body from all over and each time you take a deep breath, your confidence grows, making your presence bigger. You are in control of your energy space. Your moves will become more calculated, you'll become more aware of what comes out of your mouth and into the ears of others, and you'll allow only great thoughts to fill your mind space.

Being the rookie and the vet means understanding both the details and the overall vision of your life. It means seeing beyond yourself to consider others and how your contribution can make the world a better place. Make it a great day!

ROOT CHAKRA CHARACTERISTICS:

Feeling: Safety Color: Red Mantra: I am Crystal: Hematite

Meditation notes: How did you feel?

What thoughts/emotions came?

_____
_____
_____
_____
_____
_____
_____
_____
_____
_____
_____
_____
_____
_____
_____

MONDAY – SACRAL CHAKRA

YA FEEL ME?

"I went through every emotion with tryna pursue what I'm doing, you know what I mean? And I think what's gon' separate whoever's gon go for something, that you ain't gon' quit." – Nipsey Hussle

OVERVIEW

Monday - the first day of the work and school week gets a bad rap. Focus on the second chakra to help boost creativity energy and nurture relationships. This includes partnerships, work, and personal relationships. Monday sets the tone for the work week; how will it begin? What changes would you like to see throughout this week? We all need that extra push on Mondays, considering that it's the first day coming out of the weekend. Meditating today gives our physical and mental state of being the strength needed to put the work into wherever it needs to go today. This is also a good day for strengthening your relationships by communicating with friends and family, showing appreciation to someone, or creating new connections. Spreading your energy and good cheer is important today – it helps you, and others make the start of this week pleasant – or at least bearable.

The second day of the week – Monday is correlated to our second chakra – the sacral chakra. The sacral chakra is located about 1 inch below your navel and about 2 inches inside your body. The sacral chakra relates to our sexuality, feelings, sensuality, pleasure, passion, emotions, and creativity. Balancing our sacral chakra will allow us to release our creativity and express our authentic selves to the world. We will also understand our emotions as they come so we don't mishandle them.

We fully develop our sacral chakra's energy between the ages of 7-14. The sacral chakra holds the energy that opens our ability to feel and create. Once our basic needs are met through our balanced root chakra, we can now focus on what we like to do for pleasure and creativity through our sacral chakra.

Although today is a great day to start activities, I'm not encouraging you to get burnt out or overwhelmed. The meditation below is helping us to go through the day with bringing awareness to our physical body and our inner emotions. When we're able to bring awareness to certain parts of our body both inside and out, we'll be better able to control ourselves as a whole.

MEDITATION

As long as we're alive, our bodies are always "on" – blood is flowing, our heart is beating, pulses are pumping, hair is growing, bones are cracking…lol. What I'm trying to say is that we are always evolving and growing. When we take the time to slow down everything on the outside and actually FEEL our body running, we can become aware of areas in our bodies that we should be giving extra energy (or love) to. Our nervous system is connected to our brain, and both our mind and physical feelings (nerves) will react to situations as you take them in. When we're paying attention to our body using our body, it can be easier to take the emotions out of our heart and focus directly on relaxing and **easing** our bodies – preventing any **dis-eases** that may come.

How does your shoulders feel? What about your core area? A lot of people subconsciously contract or hold certain parts of their bodies, which over time makes it a little harder to breathe easily, and eventually that can cause health issues in our body.

When our bodies are completely still and our nerves are calm, we're able to feel our bodies in a more natural state. With this meditation, as well as anything in life, your intentions must be pure in order for it to work. The goal should be to feel your energy flowing throughout your body beyond the physical movements. Spending time in this space helps to train your brain and body on how to stay calm in times where you need it most. This preventative method to keep our bodies healthy strengthen our digestive system as well. Throughout the years, a lot of us picked up the unintentional habits of tensing up our bodies and without correcting that bad habit, it wears our bodies down prematurely.

When we use our power to control our inner selves from all the stimulants going on around us, then our aura can strengthen, and we can become more focused. We have control over what can penetrate our aura and affect us on a mental level. Feeling and getting ourselves familiar with the sensations in our body emotionally is helpful when the unexpected comes our way – big or small. We will be able to spot different areas of our body that changes physically when our emotions change. At times, when situations seem as if they are lingering in your head, it's best to take a pause and feel your emotions all the way. Sometimes you can't tiptoe around your emotions – as hard as they may be, they are real, and they are yours and they should be expressed. "Feeling yourself" in this way can help to control yourself and check yourself when things go left, so you would know how to align yourself right and go on with your life. Understand also that any feelings and thoughts that you choose to constantly experience in your body and mind, you will subconsciously search for the people, places, and things that bring you those feelings and fulfill those thoughts. Make sure to fill your mind with great thoughts, even if they seem unattainable, because your body will "feel" happy from those thoughts and bring you in the spaces where it makes you happy.

SACRAL CHAKRA CHARACTERISTICS:

Feeling: Sensuality Color: Orange Mantra: I feel Crystal: Citrine

Meditation notes: How did you feel?

What thoughts/emotions came?

_____
_____
_____
_____
_____
_____
_____
_____
_____
_____
_____
_____
_____
_____
_____

TUESDAY – SOLAR PLEXUS

BREATHE FAM

"Spirit is derive from the word "spirae", which means to breathe"
– Anthony Browder, "Nile Valley Contributions to Civilization

OVERVIEW

Tuesdays are usually overlooked and underestimated, but it's a great day to meditate so you can continue the momentum from Monday. Tuesday needs your boldness and confidence to follow through on the visions you created on Sunday and the connections you strengthened on Monday.

Tuesday can be best correlated to the solar plexus chakra. Tuesday is the 3rd day of the week. The solar plexus chakra is the 3rd chakra from the bottom, located in our abdomen, where the ribs join below our chest. We develop the solar plexus energy between the ages of 14-21.

This is the chakra that focuses its energy on balance, confidence, and self-identity – knowing who we are and what we are meant to do in the present moment and overall. Nurturing this centre of self-identity can help you maintain whatever tasks you need to work on. Remember to keep any ego thoughts out of your mind and you will sail through the rest of the week no matter what activities you have planned.

Breathing properly today will give you the inner strength to go about your day with confidence. Being confident and sure of yourself today will carry an aura of growth in you where the right people and opportunities will gravitate your way. When you are confident in yourself, your actions will show it without you having to speak.

The meditation practice below is to help with finding your body's natural breathing rhythm to balance your solar plexus. Breathing is so automatic, that we don't pay attention to whether we're doing it right or not, but what is right? Your body will be the judge of that based on your individual situation. Each moment is different and there's no 1 breathing pattern that works for all – breathing is always a work in progress. There may be emotions you've never felt before from situations you've never been through so practicing properly breathing at random moments throughout the day is necessary.

MEDITATION:

Take 4 slow deep breaths that fills your lungs with as much air as comfortably possible (like a good yawn), then slowly let it out…in…out 1…in…out…2…in…out…3…in…out…4…

On a cellular level, breathing deeply strengthens your lung tissue – think of it as mini exercises for our lungs.

Mastering your breathing to find and maintain its natural rhythm on a regular basis is a skill that needs to be practiced over time – you will not master it right away so give yourself some time and patience, but just know that if you incorporate it in your lifestyle then you're bound to become better at it. A lot of us believe that since we've been breathing our whole lives that we understand how to properly breathe. Breathing is a constant involuntarily action that will happen until the day we die – whether we do it to our benefit or detriment is up to us.

First, becoming aware of your breathing pattern at any given moment is helpful – how would you describe your breathing at this moment? Rushed? Short? Relaxed?

Secondly, we would need to put our whole attention towards the act of breathing to our natural rhythm AT THIS MOMENT (each moment will be different). Personally, I would notice that my heartbeat and breathing gives a steady rhythm whenever I breathe properly. Short breaths or long pauses in our breathing make our lungs and other organs need extra effort to make up for the lack of oxygen that's flowing.

There may be difficult or sensitive choices that need to be made throughout the day and when tensions are high, that can possibly lead to the wrong choices. Breathing deeply and properly gives our body and mind a necessary pause to collect our thoughts and our nerves before making a big decision. This keeps us aware and alert in the present moment. Breathing deeply for a few seconds can clear any cobwebs that could be stuck in our brain so we can think clearer. You can make better decisions when your mind is clear, and you won't base your reactions off emotions as much and more on logic.

When you're going through anxiety, breathing deeply helps to regulate and calm your whole body inside and outside. This is perfect time for you to appreciate and have gratitude for the ability to freely take deep breaths and fill your lungs with oxygen, because some people aren't able do so. Breathing deeply can also give you time to appreciate your life and the flow of your blood, nervous system, and mind…it brings things into perspective.

SOLAR PLEXUS CHAKRA CHARACTERISTICS:

Feeling: Confidence Color: Yellow Mantra: I do Crystal: Sunstone

Meditation notes: How did you feel?

What thoughts/emotions came?

_____
_____
_____
_____
_____
_____
_____
_____
_____
_____
_____
_____
_____
_____
_____

WEDNESDAY – HEART CHAKRA

THE GOOD GOLD RUSH

"Above all else, guard your heart, for everything you do flows from it."
– Proverbs 4:23

OVERVIEW

Since Wednesdays are in the middle of the workweek, it's an ideal day to balance and recalibrate your energy. Enough days have passed for you to reflect on what has happened, and enough days are coming up for you to adjust to what can happen. By this time, we may need to focus on our heart's energy and any emotional stuff that comes up. Perhaps something happened at work or school. Or there may be worry or fear about an upcoming event or task. Regardless of how your week started; reflecting and rebalancing your energy today can help you to control the remainder of the week.

Wednesdays are best correlated to our 4th chakra – the heart chakra. It's located in your heart area (obviously..lol). It's in the middle of your core with 3 chakras above and below it, just like Wednesday is the day in the middle of the week with 3 days above and below it. Our heart chakra is related to the energy of love - for ourselves and others as well as our love for places, things, ideas…anything that can be loved. We develop our heart chakra's energy fully between the ages of 21-28.

Love is the highest form energy that you can feel, there's no feeling higher than love – it's the most positive feeling. As great as this feeling is, a lot of people aren't receiving the full benefit of this energy. A lot of people are great at giving love, comforting, and nurturing others; but many don't know how to receive love. When our heart chakra is balanced, we can freely give AND receive love without any blockages.

This day will require you to put your "heart" into the things you do today and do them with good intentions. Intentionally expressing and pouring "love" into everything you do today and making that a practice will help you get through today and beyond. When you pour love, or your heart into your daily activities, you're putting your positive energy into them intentionally, you're not just letting the day's activities happen by chance. On Wednesdays, we need that extra internal push that comes from meditating to balancing our heart chakra. When your heart is in a good space, it can start to intuitively guide you towards the life you want, or at least the moments you want, which leads to days, weeks, years, and a life you want.

The purpose of this meditation is to help you realize the importance of your heart's energy. When you're feeling good, your heart feels good – and call it whatever you want, but there's something happening in your heart that will bring more good things to you. When we are doing things "with a cheerful heart", the power behind your cheerful heart will propel whatever it is you're doing. Projecting good energy from your heart releases an aura that others can feel with their heart, and deeper communication can happen between the two.

MEDITATION

One of the most important organs in our body is our heart, it's the pulse of our life. This life-giving organ pumps and recirculates the blood that flows throughout your body every second of every day. It's amazing that our heart is a natural pumping system for our blood. Of course, what we eat and how we treat our body plays a major role in the health of our heart and body, but I believe FEELING good feelings with our heart holds just as much weight when developing a healthy heart.

Whether good or bad - whenever you're feeling an extreme emotion from something being said or done, physically your heart tends to beat more intense. Whether you're extremely happy, extremely angry, or extremely fearful…the intensity of your heart is the same, just with different emotions attached to them.

I believe the quality of our life is partly determined by how intentional our hearts are, or how much love we give throughout the days. When you feel good in your heart and heighten those feelings, your presence alone will bless others and make them feel good because you're giving those good feelings to everyone you interact with. When you feel bad, not only are you giving those bad feelings to others, but the tension causes your nerves and cells to contract, the vital chemical production in your body changes, your blood vessels contract, and your breathing becomes shallow, all of which reduces the health in your organs and your entire body. Disease is simply the result of a body's not being at ease over a long period of time, because of negative feelings like stress, worry, and fear.

Overall, how does your heart feel right now? Happy? Content? Relaxed? Stressed? I believe when you strengthen your heart with great thoughts/memories/dreams periodically, your aura will start to attract those things that bring happiness and meaning in your life. The time you spend meditating gives your heart and mind a chance to "pump" out the happy chemical our body craves - endorphins – which I call the good gold rush! Our bodies naturally erupt this chemical from within only when we're feeling good, and that chemical flows throughout our body. Imagine the feeling you would get if you saw a postcard in the mail from your childhood best friend that you haven't heard from in years. All types of emotions like gratitude, love, happiness, appreciation, etc will rush out of you. Feeling intense bursts of happiness and joy periodically is good for your health – even when things like that aren't happening. Similar to a storehouse of medicine, this internal rush delivers ease and comfort in your body – preventing any disease that could be accumulating. The "good gold rush" going all up and through your body serves as your personal protection throughout the day. You have that ability to cultivate that power whenever you need it.

Of course, we know that it's impossible to feel great every second of the day - there will be bad times and there will be horrible days. Sometimes, our minds is in a completely different space and can't cooperate with anything that's going on. When that happens, acknowledge and feel those emotions fully…then try to understand those emotions and where it's coming from.

Also, stopping yourself throughout the day to check in with yourself on the type of "rush" your body is having can save you from getting lost in your thoughts. Is it a good rush? Bad rush? Okay rush?

Lastly, understand that feelings and emotions are real, and they are in constant motion. Some feelings are easy to understand and explain, while other feelings are better "felt" and cannot be understood or explained. Humans are dynamic with a lot of things going on at once, so it's likely that you're feeling a combination of feelings depending on where your thoughts are. Having the ability to work with our emotions instead of them working us can help you cope with yourself and others peacefully.

HEART CHAKRA CHARACTERISTICS:

Feeling: Love Color: Green Mantra: I love Crystal: Rose quartz

Meditation notes: How did you feel? What thoughts came to mind?

_____
_____
_____
_____
_____
_____
_____
_____
_____
_____
_____
_____
_____
_____
_____
_____
_____

THURSDAY – THROAT CHAKRA

SAY WHAT YOU MEAN AND MEAN WHAT YOU SAY

They say conversation, rule a nation, I can tell But I can never right my wrongs 'less I write it down for real" – Kendrick Lamar

OVERVIEW

Work and school involve a lot of communication, so Thursday is a good day to work on any issues you need to express and be open to receiving information as you head towards the end of the week. This is also a great day for tightening up your communication with yourself and others before the weekend starts. Release what you cannot say or give voice to the things that you should say today.

Building yourself up by affirming, or verbally acknowledging your best qualities can propel you forward on how great your weekend can turn out to be. Thursday can be seen as a "wrap up" day for the week so that the weekend can go smoothly. This will be a good day for verbalizing any goals you'd like to accomplish during the weekend – whether it be relaxing, taking a small trip, or handling some business. This is also a good day to give others the energy boost they may need from your energy, or most important – from your words - as the week closes out by speaking affirmations to them.

It's natural for us not to always be in the best mood to speak great things to ourselves or feel our best. Life happens, and sometimes life happens hard. For down-times like those, and you can't shake it off, then you just need to face it.

Sometimes our mind can take us to a dark place without our permission, and if we ignore or try to hide it, we can self-destruct. You may have to sit in those emotions and feel them all the way in order to understand them (and yourself) better and possibly heal from the situation.

There may be times where you feel a dark cloud over you, and you don't know why. We may have to be strategic and allow our mind to soak in great things. We have access to an abundance of information we can watch, listen to, or read about that can give us the encouragement we need.

We don't have to do all the mental work to get ourselves out of a funk sometimes if it's not necessary. You can just sit back and play some nice music or a motivational speech/interview in the background and soak in whatever resonates.

When you can use the power of words to saturate yourself with thoughts that can raise your vibrations…you will gain a power that you can use at will. You can change your emotions better when you're able to acknowledge those emotions and understand why they're there.

The chakra that correlates with Thursday is our throat chakra – which is related to how we communicate with ourselves and others. It's located in the throat area, and we fully develop this chakra between the ages of 28-35.

The right words can bring on the feelings that gets you excited and inspired. Great words and a great conversation between people can be energizing and can change lives.

It stimulates you when you have a great conversation with someone. On the other hand, the wrong words or a bad conversation can bring destruction, harm, and lifelong problems.

MEDITATION

Words matter. They have the power to create things into existence and influence others. What you say to yourself (and others) is important because it is heard first in your mind before comes out of your mouth.

Saying positive things about yourself and to yourself helps your subconscious form the image of who you desire to be (which will be a lifelong project because we are always growing and experiencing different things). The words and thoughts you have with yourself matter the most because each time you say or think something, that thought is impressed in your brain once more.

Similar to folding a piece of paper numerous times the same way – that impression will become deeper and will eventually have a permanent place in your mind and lifestyle. Saying and thinking great things to yourself will prime your body for the day because you're better able to see yourself and move as the person who fits your affirmations.

When you combine your belief, or faith in your affirmations with great emotions about them, the chances of that affirmation manifesting will grow, and you will realize you can do amazing things.

It would be great if we all understood our place and purpose on earth, but life doesn't give us those instructions – we are free to do whatever we want to do, and a lot of us don't know what to do, so most times, we do the wrong things.

I believe that every single person has a purpose or contribution on earth, and it comes in the form of what we naturally love to do Everyone has those basic needs: to live comfortably, be healthy, and have good relationships, but each person also has a unique set of needs and desires they want to fulfill that's different than everyone else.

When we find time to do those things we naturally love to do, we can better understand which direction our life should go. When we know what our purpose is in life, we can better see and speak ourselves into thriving within that space.

Sometimes you know exactly what you need to say to yourself for the words to genuinely penetrate your soul to create the change or growth you need. Talk to yourself as if you are your own mentor and have those hard conversations with yourself. Go deep, then go deeper – you can NEVER go too deep. Express to yourself how much you care about your well-being and reassure yourself that you will get through any obstacle.

THROAT CHAKRA CHARACTERISTICS:

Feeling: Self-esteem Color: Blue Mantra: I speak Crystal: Sodalite

Meditation notes: How did you feel?

What thoughts/emotions came?

FRIDAY – THIRD EYE CHAKRA

INNER(G)

"My two eyes saw your third eye from across the room; I can see your soul babe and I think you're my soul mate" – Big Krit

OVERVIEW

Fridays start the weekend, and for most people, it's time to relax and unwind. Whether you're off work and focusing on home or school life, watching a movie, or just want to go out and have a good time – Friday is usually the day where you want to make that happen, while still tending to what you HAVE to do. As we move into the weekend there is a shift in perspective. By working with your intuitive center, you can focus and trust what guides you.

Since you're usually open to more choices of things to do on Fridays, you may be tempted to do things you may not need to do or isn't for your best interest. Listening to your inner (G)angsta AKA your intuition, is imperative for guiding you today (and any other day). Your inner(G) is the wise voice in your head who's bold enough to speak the truth and tell you what you need to hear, whether you like it or not.

Your 3rd eye chakra is the chakra that best correlates with Friday's energy and it's all about focusing on your intuition – that voice of reason that warns you and helps you to feel out the world and everything in it. We develop our third eye chakra between the ages of 35-42.

Meditating with a focus on this chakra can help you to make better choices throughout the day and keep you protected from any harm that comes in many forms.

You're able to sense people's true intentions and listen beyond the words they're saying. You will be able to step into a room and FEEL if something isn't right and that will be enough reason for you to leave soon. Your 3rd eye can see beyond your regular 2 eyes and it brings awareness to situations that are brewing in the background without you consciously knowing or seeing it.

You need protection from your inner(g) to function in your day-to-day life. When your 3rd eye chakra is not balanced, it's hard to spot danger when it's around and that can lead to trouble for you and others. Your ability to "read the room" or feel the energy of the space may be hindered without you tapping into your intuition.

MEDITATION

A lot of us have an ideal version of who we want to be – it's human nature to want to see ourselves at our best. It's okay to be both satisfied with where you're at in life AND still want more – there's more out there. It can be frustrating when we feel that we are not living up to our fullest potential because we know we are full of potential.

We sometimes get caught up on our failures, or attempts at life, comparing our current selves to who we think we SHOULD be and becoming disappointed knowing we can do and be better. This is where it's a good practice to tap into the emotional state you would be in IF all your goals are unfolding, and life is going your way. The excitement in your heart will raise your energy towards becoming that evolved version of yourself.

Although you want to be great in every aspect of your life, humble yourself enough to know you're a normal human who will do normal human things. Don't expect perfection, just effort and progression. Also know that you have the potential to do normal things in a great way. When you listen to your inner(G), those normal things you do can be done in a great way.

What normal things could you do greatly? Communicate? Cook? Rest/

relax? If you can clearly visualize the kind of person you aspire to be, you will be aware of what needs to shift within your character to get you closer to that person.

That version of you exists because you birthed that possibility of yourself (in your mind) and you can feel that energy. We can appreciate the power our imagination has on our excitement and happiness of what we CAN be. Put your energy towards your inner(G) and see what changes you notice within yourself when you're in different situations.

Does your inner(G) feel rushed with some people? Does it calm down with others? Have you felt anxiety or tension in a room? Have you felt comfort and warmth in other rooms? Your third eye will tell you exactly what you need to know without verbalizing anything. When your thoughts become calmer over time with meditation, your inner(G) becomes louder and clearer.

Your inner(G) has no filter. It doesn't care how your feelings are about a situation. No amount of rationalizing or logic will matter when your inner(G) kicks in. Your inner(G) knows what's right and what's wrong and will let you know before your brain comprehends it. Letting go and trusting in your inner(G) will help you to move throughout your days with ease.

THIRD EYE CHAKRA CHARACTERISTICS:

Feeling: Intuitive Color: Purple Mantra: I know Crystal: Amethyst

Meditation notes: How did you feel?

What thoughts/emotions came?

_____
_____
_____
_____
_____
_____
_____
_____
_____
_____
_____
_____
_____
_____
_____
_____
_____

SATURDAY – CROWN CHAKRA

REMEMBER THE TIME

"Heavy is the head that chose to wear the crown
To whom is given much is required now" – Kendrick Lamar

OVERVIEW

The last day of the week – Saturday, gives us time to renew our connection with our Source. This is our time to reconnect with home life, family, friends, and ourselves. Saturdays are also good days for rest and relaxation, the Sabbath day – this day brings us back mentally and physically "home" after a workweek of doing things.

Saturdays are good days to reflect on all the events that happened this past week, whether good or bad. Maybe certain connections and conversations strike out as important and need to be followed up on , or you may have realized you need to cut some ties with certain people, things, or habits, which is fine as well. This week has for sure taught you lessons, intentionally or unintentionally, but it's up to you to figure out what those lessons are and what to take from them.

The crown chakra is the last of our seven main chakras and it has many correlations to Saturday. The crown chakra is located right above our head, the last chakra starting from the root and its mantra is "I am". We fully develop our crown chakra's energy between the ages of 43-49. The crown chakra represents bringing everything together and connecting to our source.

The crown chakra energy focuses on who we truly are when we take away all the layers that have been placed on us throughout the years. It's self-knowledge, stripping of the ego. This chakra represents our true essence, it's the energy within us that knows our true purpose and that we are here for a reason.

MEDITATION

Who are you? After everything is said and done, what do you represent? What do you stand for? After all what you've been through to make it this far, where is your heart at? We all have a story – some people embrace it while others suppress it and try to forget it. "Embracing it" doesn't mean professing to the world all your flaws, but rather knowing and accepting that there has been good and bad in your life that contributes to who you are.

While meditating today, take some time to think about who you are as a whole – how you are as a parent, child, friend, employee, etc. Dig deeper into how your upbringing affected who you are as a person and how it has impacted your life and others. Whether good or bad, everything that has happened in your life contributes to who you are. If your thoughts take you to some undesirable events in your life while you meditate – stay there – it's resurfacing for a reason…that's how you embrace and eventually accept it.

It's amazing that we have this wonderful gift to remember, reflect, and assess our lives, which is powerful for us. This is one of our gifts that separates us from most animals. I don't believe a cat or a dog reflects over where their life has been or where it's going in a philosophical way…they live off of instinct and survival.

A lot of us do not realize the importance of periodically taking a step back from our busy lives to remember our growth and the lessons that life has taught us. We can look back on our lives with wisdom, and know that we are a better, more learned version of who we once were. Although you've came a long way, take time to think about all of the untapped potential that has yet to be expressed to yourself and others so far.

Currently, you are the wisest you have ever been in your life. Good or bad…up to this moment, you have experienced and know more than what you knew a year ago, a month ago, a week ago, even an hour ago. We are constantly learning new things whether we're aware of it or not – our growth is inevitable.

On the flip side, we also must take into consideration that no matter how learned or wise we may become, we have yet to experience everything that life has to offer. That is the beauty of life - there is basically no limit to what we can learn and do.

We are always going to be students in life, but we choose what we pour our energy into & want to learn from. We are always going through new situations and growth and challenges that are the accumulation of what we have already gone through.

Some things in life come at us from such an unexpected angle that we were never prepared for. That's why we need to equip ourselves with the strength of meditation to fight these battles that we were not prepared for when they come. There is a certain type of power that we have to tap into that we can't get from any outside energy. That power comes from remembering who you were as you continuously grow through your stages of life.

CROWN CHAKRA CHARACTERISTICS:

Feeling: Self-knowledge Color: White Mantra: I understand

Crystal: Clear Quartz Meditation notes: How did you feel?

What thoughts/emotions came?

_____

_____

_____

_____

_____

_____

_____

_____

_____

_____

_____

_____

_____

_____

_____

_____

CONCLUSION

"Young carter go faster go further go farther, is that not why we came and if not, then why bother" – Jay Z

We are at a time in life where more people are understanding the importance of meditation on a collective level and what it can also do in our individual lives. Just think of how easier life can be if we choose to meditate daily. We can think clearly, address situations as they come, work through our emotions, and have enough high vibrations to encourage others who may need it. It starts with someone taking those actions one by one, so why not be one of them?

A lot of people have the desire to meditate but claim to never have the time or energy. I am sorry to say, but that's a personal accountability issue I can't help you out with. I can however help you out with analogies and stories to think about once you've made the decision to meditate, but anything before that is out of my control. No one will come into your house and convince you to meditate everyday – it must be something that you intentionally want to do. Using other resources such as (more) books, YouTube, online courses, and just old-fashioned practicing will help build the habit. Everyone's vibe and learning style is different, so the specific things that works for me, may not work for you, but the overall goal is the same – different roads leading to the same destination. We must hold ourselves accountable and understand that if we're not putting our time and energy into something…anything, then it's not going to get better, PERIOD.

For me, facing the realities of being a single black mother, I saw that meditation is one of the few things that can keep me sane amid living within my demographics in one of the most segregated cities in America (Milwaukee, WI). I understood that down the line, I would eventually become better at meditation and my body and mind will fall in place on demand. I know that there are always going to be deeper feelings and emotions that I can go into when meditating. Everything you do has to be backed up with the right intentions. When we are doing things "with a cheerful heart" as they say, the power behind that "cheerful heart" will propel whatever it is you're doing.

I hope this booklet gave you good insights into different thoughts that you can focus on and that you can use this as a resource for years to come. Read it as many times as you need to grasp the concepts. There are MANY different ways to meditate, and no one is right or wrong… there's just a groove that you have to find that fits you individually. It'll be hard as hell to expect us to be able to shut down EVERY thought that's going on, but it is possible to have a better control of the thoughts that passes by your mind. Strengthening the flow of your thoughts will take time and practice, just like anything else that you want to get better at. We are living in a fast paced, information driven society and now we are seeing the effects of what happens when we don't slow down and become aware and appreciate of the little things individually and collectively.

Hopefully you understand a little more about chakras and how they relate to our everyday life. I wanted to touch on the surface of chakras and give a basic overview of them, but there is an abundance of information available to learn more. I'm definitely not an expert but I understand enough.

There can be value found in each day of the week…there's not one day more important than the other. Each of these meditations doesn't have to be practiced on the specific day that it's under, it's just a way to get your body and mind relaxed and focused for the meditation.

As I mentioned in the beginning of this book; life is hard for every one.

We all have our different cards that has been dealt to us, and although they vary, they are just as mixed up as the next person's cards. When we meditate, we learn how to organize our messy cards to at least have it in order.

The great thing about meditation is that you don't need any fancy equipment or tools to begin. Your attention is the most important tool that's needed for an effective meditation. Hopefully you've already practiced a few times by now, but if not, you will realize how simple it is.

This free service to yourself has the potential to change your life and the lives of others around you. When others see the change within you, without you having to announce it, that will inspire them to follow the path.

I'm so grateful that you decided to give this book a try. Learning something new after we're grown is difficult, so I commend you for taking that step. However, your journey has just begun.

There is so much more to explore and experience with meditation that it'll send you out of this world. Please share this book with someone if you find it helpful or keep this handy if ever you need a quick push when things are going haywire.

With Love,

Celeste M

ACKNOWLEDGMENTS:

I want to first thank God/Universe/Creator/Higher Power for the ideas and momentum brought to me so I can bring this book to you. A good friend of mine, G has been a great inspiration and push for me to stay consistent in creating his book, and to help me realize that we're living in a time where this world is coming back to an understanding and appreciation for meditation - without his excitement and wise insight, this book probably would've stayed an idea. Tone has been a great supporter in everything I do from the start, and as with everything else, I appreciate the input and him being a crutch when I needed it. All my friends and family who encouraged me along the way or helped me to tweak some parts and provided constructive criticism deserve my thanks and gratitude. I'm grateful for all the readers and supporters who will utilize this book and the techniques to gain inner strength for a better life within.

DEDICATION:

I dedicate this book to whoever's striving to find their inner peace amidst all the craziness going on - regardless of if they admit it/know it or not. A lot of people say they are okay because it sounds good verbally, but deep down inside, we are all battling different levels of depression that are hidden and slowly eating away at us if we allow it. I hope this book will allow you and me to open up and strive to become full again... that journey is much better.

www.ingramcontent.com/pod-product-compliance
Lightning Source LLC
Chambersburg PA
CBHW031207090426
42736CB00009B/818